Table of Co

Copyright

Preface

"To be beautiful means to be yourself.
You don't need to be accepted by others.
You just need to accept yourself."
— Thich Nhat Hanh

Introduction

William Shakespeare once said, "Eyes are the windows to your soul". Well honey, if that's true; I want my 'windows' to be absolutely fabulous and beautifully decorated!

Eye makeup is nothing new. It has a history that stretches as far back as 10,000 BC where Egyptian women and men would line their eyes and eyebrows with Kohl made from almonds, ash, copper and other compound minerals. It was seen as not only fashionable, but believed to decrease the glare of the sun.

In 11th century Japan, girls would decorate their eyes with an eye shadow concoction made from rice flour, crushed flower petals and bird dropping (gross huh?).

And who can forget the 1960's where the first supermodel, Twiggy, popularized the bright eye shadow look paired with bold lashes and intense eyeliner.

It's an understatement to say eye makeup is as versatile as the history behind it. Eye shadows come in thousands of shades, textures and finishes. Eyebrows can be accentuated with pencil, power, wax, gel and even markers. And let's not even get started on mascara, with the many different mascara wands and looks!

So before we get super deep into the eye makeup, let me introduce myself! I'm Breonna Queen Lewis, although most know me simply as Breonna Queen. I am a makeup artist, beauty educator, speaker, and business owner of a fabulous lipstick line called *Queenie Skin & Cosmetics.* My beauty YouTube Channel has thousands of subscribers and millions of views and my work has been featured in popular blogs. I wrote this book series, Just Face It!, to give in-depth information on makeup so no matter your makeup level; you can understand cosmetics and how to achieve your desired look.

If you have not checked out my first book of this series, JUST *FACE IT!: A makeup guide for Skincare and Foundation*, I seriously urge you to check it out since it provides in-depth information on building your skin regime for healthy, beautiful, pimple-free skin (which is the most important first step to any makeup look!).

So now let's get started on eye makeup! Say hello to finally perfecting that winged liner and kiss those failed smoky eye attempts goodbye.

Eyebrows

Ask a makeup artist how important eyebrows are on a scale from to 1 to 10 and I'm sure she will say 15. Eyebrows are extremely important as they not only prevent sweat and dirt from falling into your eye socket, but they also help frame your face and complete your look. Don't believe me? Google, "celebrities without eyebrows" and see how important eyebrows play in complimenting your face.

The shape of your eyebrows can alter the entire look of your face, so be sure you are grooming them to go with the natural shape of your face. Brow shaping isn't rocket science but perfecting can take practice. When I first started grooming my eyebrows, I tweezed them pencil thin. I can laugh about it now but when I look at old pictures, I cringe as how harsh they made my face appear. Listen, I'm telling you this so you don't fall victim to the over plucked brows (or perhaps never be the victim again!).

A lot of women often ask me how to find the natural shape of their brows and honestly, you just have to look at your eyebrows. Is there an arch? Is there a high arch?
If you are suffering from overly plucked eyebrows and can't really tell, I recommend looking at a picture of you when you were a child. What was your arch like as a child?

As a child, I had a soft curved arch. I still have a soft curved arch; it's just more defined now!

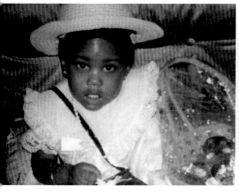
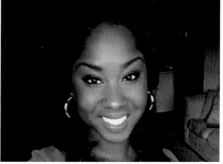

Another example is Beyoncé. She had a high arch as a baby and still has a high arch (except now, it's more defined!)

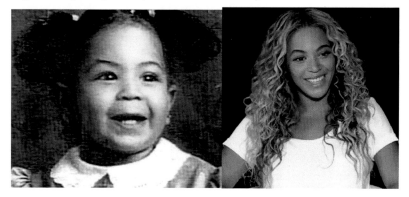

Brow Shaping

There are 3 key points to your eyebrows:

1.   The Starting Point (a)

The starting point is where your eyebrows begin. Eyebrows should start perpendicular to the inner corners of your eye.

2.   The Arch (b)

the arch is the highest point of your eyebrows. Generally arches should be parallel to the outside corner of your iris; however, some people don't have an arch at all.

3.   The Ending point (c)

The ending point is pretty self-explanative. However, just to be clear it's where the eyebrow ends. The end of the brow point should be at a 45-degree angle from the outside end of the eye. Usually eyebrows thin out at the end.

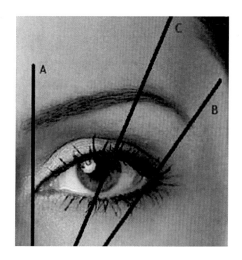

Different Eyebrow Shapes

There are lots of variations to eyebrow shapes but generally there are 4 different categories eyebrow shapes fall into:

1.   Round

Rounded eyebrows generally have a small to medium arch and work best for softening defined facial angles. They have no angles and are curved.

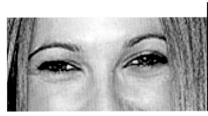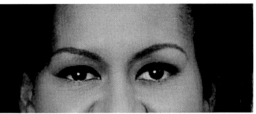

2.   Curved

The eyebrow has a soft curve that generally follows the shape of the eyelid The angle is not sharp

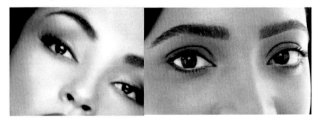

3.   Arch

prominent angles that clearly have a sharp arch. The degree of archness varies as you can have a soft arch or a high arch.

High Arch and a Low Arch:

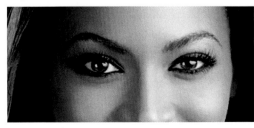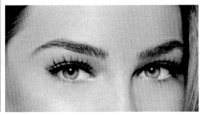

4.   Flat (straight)

Very little arch and angle, eyebrow mostly runs in a straight line.

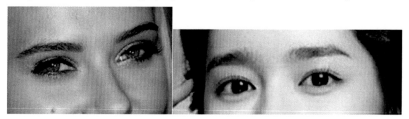

Tips:

- If you have small eyes, keep your eyebrow arch low (close to the eyes) which will make your eyes appear larger.

- If you have big eyes, keep your eyebrow arch high (far from eyes) which will create an illusion of smaller eyes.

Different Methods for filling in eyebrows

Eyebrows don't always grow in the same thickness. When eyebrows are sparse, fill them in! However, practice and patience is key! Too much eyebrow filling can have you looking like Bert from Sesame Street! Too little and you may as well not even apply any.

1. Eyebrow Gel

Fills eyebrows as well as keeps your eyebrow hair in place.

Can be used alone or after applying pencil to eyebrows to "soften" the look and keep the hairs in place. Clear eyebrow gel will keep unruly eyebrow hairs in place. Tinted eyebrow gel will fill in the brows as well brush the brow hairs into a certain place.

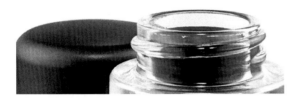

2. Eyebrow Pencil

helps to fill in brows and shape them. I recommend using quick short pencil stroke as that mimics hair.

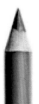 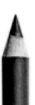 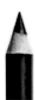

3. Eyebrow Tinting

the same way you tint your hair on your head, you can tint your eyebrows! Eyebrow tinting usually consist of darkening the eyebrows so they appear more apparent and fuller on the face. Just be careful not to tint black as it can appear too harsh on the face!

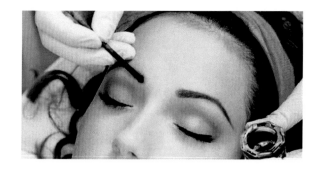

4.   Eyebrow Powder

A powdered formula to fill in and shape brows. Generally less harsh than pencil. Can be used after applying pencil to give a softer look to brows or to give a more natural look to brows.

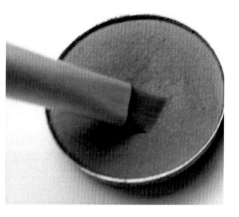

How to fill in your eyebrows

1. Start with clean brows and brush brows with a spoolie in an upward motion going from front to the end of your brow

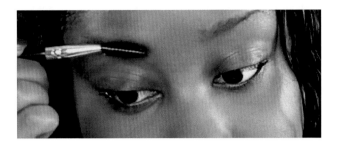 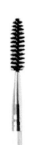

2. Using short dash strokes to mimic hair, softly filling in sparse areas with your pencil, gel or powder. Make sure the color matches your natural hairs. I like to use a pencil to fill in my brows and then go over that with a powder.

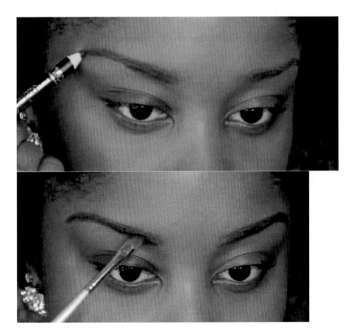

3. Brush through the brows again to blend out any color so the brows don't look harsh

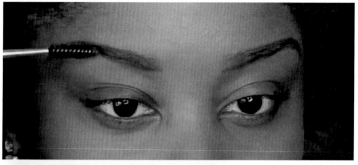

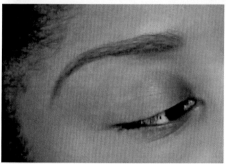

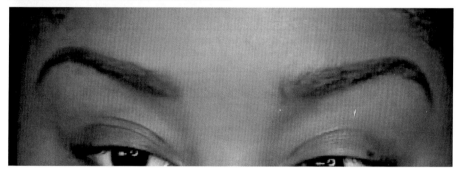

BONUS: You can apply concealer (1-2 shades lighter than you) around your eyebrows to give an instant clean look to your brows. Take a concealer brush and apply it to the lower brow bone. You can also apply the foundation at the top but be sure it's a color similar to your complexion (and not too light). Blend out and *voila*!

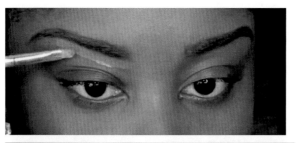

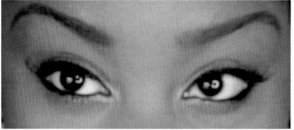

So now that we have quickly covered the basics of eyebrows, let's move on to one of the most popular and dreaded areas of makeup: eye shadow!

Eye Shadow Primer and Base

Eye shadow Primer and Eye shadow base are actually two completely different things although some products can serve as both! *Eye shadow primer* is used to prevent creasing and fading as well as improve longevity of shadows. However, *eye shadow base* is used to intensity color and help powder eye shadows adhere better to the eyelids. These days, a lot of products are both eye shadow primers and an eye shadow base to help minimize work. In this section, I will combine the two since they are applied the same way and reap similar benefits. Just remember that if it's clear, it's a probably just a primer (which it should say on the label). If it's a thick consistency with some color to it, it's a base.

Benefits of Eye shadow Primer and Base:

Eye shadow Primer is used to coat your eyelids before applying eye shadow. Some Benefits of using an eye shadow primer:

- Prevent or decrease eye shadow from creasing and smudging
- Allow a smooth canvas to apply/blend shadows
- Improve the longevity of your eye shadow
- Brighten your eye shadow
- Even skin tone, cover visible veins

How to apply eye shadow base

You can prime your eyelids by applying a concealer, an eye shadow base (such as a creamy eye shadow) or use an eye shadow primer which is created specifically for priming lids!

1. Take a small amount of primer/base and apply onto a clean eyelid with your fingers or eye shadow brush. Apply to your entire lid and a little above your crease. You also want to make sure you apply as close to your lash line as possible. Be sure to blend evenly and only apply a fine layer (you don't want to apply too much which will cause a thick cake build-up).

2. Allow the eye shadow primer and/or base to set/dry on your lid. (No longer than 2 minutes)

3. Apply eye shadow on top

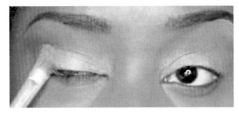

Eye shadows

I remember the first eye shadow palette I ever purchased. It was a 12 eye shadow palette from Claire's that had an assortment of shimmer-sheer shadows. I would take the lime green (my favorite eye shadow color at the time) and pack it on my eyelid. I would then top it off with a thick line of liquid eyeliner and a few coats of mascara. Blending wasn't as popular back then so my 15 year old self truly felt I was the crème de la crème with my shimmery lime green eye shadow and high shine matching lip-gloss. Oh, how times have changed. Thank goodness.

Types of Eye shadows

1.   Pressed

One of the most popular types of eye shadows. Pressed into a dry solid form. Less messy and can come in a single or multiple forms such as a palette or quad. Easily Bendable

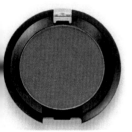

2.   Loose Powder/Pigment

Loose powder can be used with fingers, dry brush, wet brush or a sponge. Loose powder can be messy as the powders are well, duh, loose. Easily Blendable.

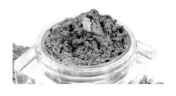

3.   Cream/Gel

can be used alone or as an eye shadow base. Can be in a jar or pencil form. Generally water-proof but can be difficult to blend due to the texture Has a shorter shelf/storage life due to the moisture.

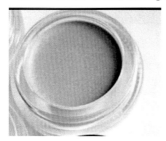

4.   Liquid

Similar to the cream and gel eye shadows, however, are in a liquid form. Does not blend as easily as powder shadows due to liquid/gel having faster drying times. Has a tendency to dry out due to the moisture level but can generally be long-lasting and smudge-proof when applied to the eye (once dried). Great as an eye shadow base.

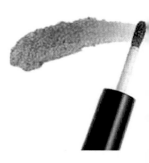

5.   Baked

Eye shadow that is "baked" into form, instead of pressed into form. Smooth texture and can be used wet or dry which allow for 2 different looks to be achieve with one single eye shadow. Less messy

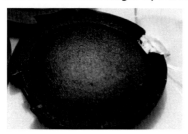

Types of Eye shadow Finishes

1. Matte Eye shadow

Does not reflect light. No shine, glitter or frost. Can also be used for contouring, eyebrow powder and blushes. However, can be chalky (dry, powdery)

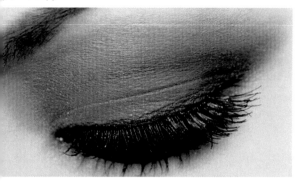

2. Satin Eye shadow

Mimics the fabric satin. Soft sheen/shimmer that allows the skin to show through. It's between matte and frost and tends to be a popular for highlight

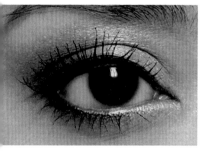

3. Pearl/ Frost

Contains reflecting particles that produce a "pearl" effect. Iridescent and generally a subtle shimmer or a high-shine. Not recommended for mature skin as it can accentuate flaws in skin such as wrinkles.

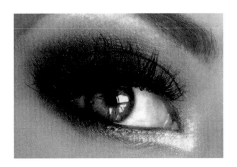

4. Glitter eye shadow:

Glitter mixed into the shadow. Usually needs an eye shadow base and should be packed on the lid (vs. sweeping) to prevent eye shadow fall-out. Can be a matte eye shadow with glitter or any shimmer finish shadow with glitter.

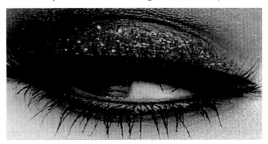

5. Metallic eye shadow:

A finish similar to metal (think foil, silver, gold, and bronze). Great for creating intense looks for nightwear. This type is eye shadow is not recommended for people with mature skin as it can highlight wrinkles.

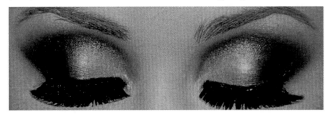

Eye Spacing Tips

To determine which eye shape spacing category you might fall into, look at the space in between your eyes. If the space between your eyes is smaller than the length of one eye, you have <u>close set eyes</u>. If its winder, you had <u>wide set eyes</u>. Here are a few tips depending on the spacing of your eyes:

Close set eyes:

Refrain from applying dark colors on your tear duct as this can make your eyes appear even closer together. The key is you want balance! Dark eye shadows should remain on your outer V and end of the eyes. Highlighting the inner corner of your eyes with a light shimmer/pear eye shadow also works great at creating a visual distance appearance. Also don't line your bottom lid all the way. Try lining your waterline ¾ of the way or adding a lighter color to the waterline (as oppose to dark brown).

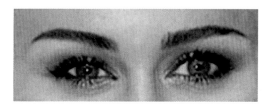

Wide set eyes:

 If you feel your eyes are too far apart, one trick to make them look closer is to apply dark shadows closer to your tear ducts. You also want to make sure you keep your eyebrows short. Extending your eyebrows can cause your face and eyes to look further apart.

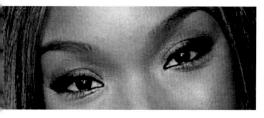

Normal: If you space between your eyes is equal then you have "normal" spacing eyes (whatever that means). I hate the term "normal" because it implies that if you have wide set or close set eyes then you are not normal and some kind of freakish weird alien (which is not true). However, if the spacing between your eyes tends to be balanced 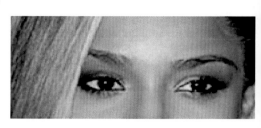 then you can play around with different colors in your tear-ducts and outer-v.

Eye shadow Placement

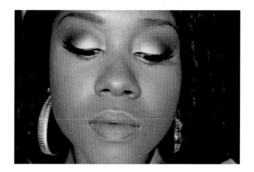

When referring to placing eye shadows on your eye, we break it into 3 sections:

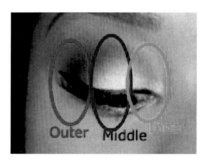

- **Inner**: Closest section your nose
- **Middle**: Center of your eye
- **Outer**: Closest to your ear

Crease: where your eye folds (eye socket). *Note: some people have a defined crease where others don't.* Generally, adding a dark color to your crease with add depth and dimension (great for those sultry looks).

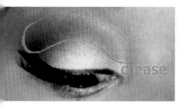

Tear duct: inner most point of the eye (closest to the nose). Appling a light color to this area works as a great highlight as it helps to brighten the eye and add dimension to a look.

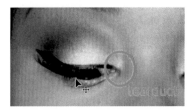

Brow bone: the bone right below your right eyebrow

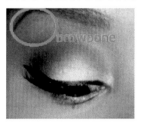

Waterline: inner rim of your lash line. When you line your waterline, its call tight-lining.

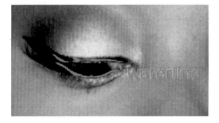

Lash line: right along the lash line.

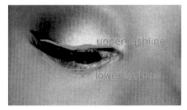

Outer: V: Area at the outermost corner of your eye (furthest away from your nose). Generally, shaped like a sideways 'V' (hence the name 'out-v') but can also be shaped like the letter 'c' for a softer look.

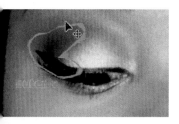

Okay, now try to name each placement illustrated by a different color!

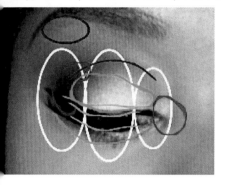

Tips

- Pack on Eye shadows: When applying eye shadow, I HIGHLY recommend investing in great eye brushes. I know the world of makeup brushes can be overwhelming but I do recommend you invest in at least an eye shadow brush; a blending brush and smudge brush (skip to the section below for the details on brushes). Anyway, when applying eye shadow you want to "pack" the eye shadows on. Packing the eye shadows on (vs. rubbing the eye shadow on your lid) allows you to get the best color pay-off and the least amount of eye shadow fall-out. You want to apply your primer and/or base first. Then you want to pack on your eye shadows.

- Light eye shadow VS Dark Eye shadow Colors: Remember the golden rule: light colors emphasize and dark colors deemphasize. When you apply a light color, you are bringing that area forward. When you apply a dark color, you are giving that area depth and receding it. Additionally, a mid-tone (medium) color will allow you to add shape without too much depth or focus.

Eye shadow Looks:

Basic Eye look:

This eye shadow look is super basic and great for beginners and those who do not want to spend a lot of time in front of the mirror. Also great if you do not have a lot of makeup brushes. This look only needs two eye shadow colors (a light color and dark color).

1. Take a light eye shadow and apply to your inner and center lid
2. Take a dark eye shadow and apply to the outer lid of your eye. *For a more seamless look, blend the line between the light eye shadow and the dark eye shadow with a fluffy blending brush*
3. Apply Eyeliner (optional but recommended!) and mascara!

Smoky eye:

This eye shadow looks includes 4 colors: the lightest eye shadow color (tear duct and lid), Medium Color eye shadow (crease), your transition color and a dark color eye shadow (outer-v). This is a great eye shadow rule for Smoky eye and you can play around with colors and textures!

1. Apply an eye shadow base

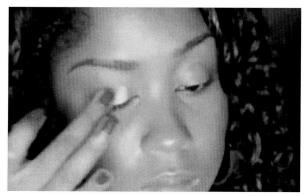

2. Take your face powder or eye shadow similar to your complexion and lightly sweep it above your crease (we call this a transition color)

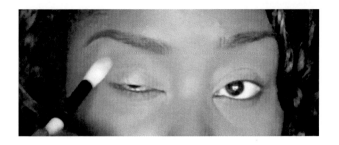

3. Take a light shimmer eye shadow (satin and shimmer for a nice pop or matte for emphasis) and apply to your tear ducts and to your lid completely.

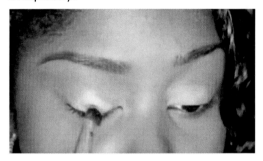

4. Take the medium color eye shadow and apply a little higher than your crease. Blend out with a fluffy brush

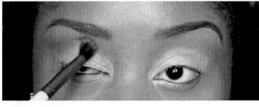

5. Take the darkest color eye shadow and apply to your outer v.

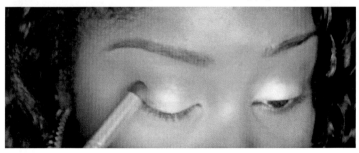

6. Blend out any harsh edges. Apply eyeliner and mascara (or lashes!)

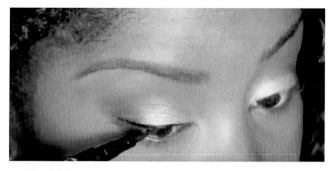

7. Wa-lah!

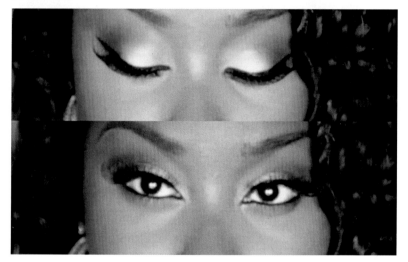

Creased Defined Smoky eye:

This eye shadow looks includes 4 colors: the lightest eye shadow color (tear duct), light eye shadow color (eyelid), Medium Color eye shadow (crease) and dark color eye shadow (outer-v). This is a great eye shadow rule for Smoky eye and you can play around with colors and textures!

7. Apply an eye shadow base

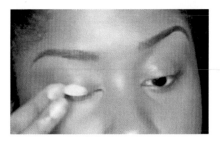

8. Take a light shimmer eye shadow (satin and shimmer for a nice pop or matte for emphasis) and apply to your tear ducts and lid.

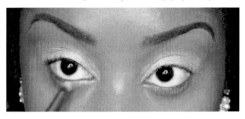

9. Take the medium color eye shadow and apply a little higher than your crease. For a more natural look, try a shadow that's similar to your complexion (this is called a transition color). For a bolder look, apply shadow 1-2 shades darker than your complexion. You'll want to apply this eye shadow to your cream with a blending brush. For a super Smoky eye, I recommend blending out the harsh line of the transition color with your fluffy brush

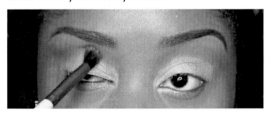

10. Take the darkest color eye shadow and apply that directly on your crease. For a smokier eye, I recommend blending out with a fluffy brush.

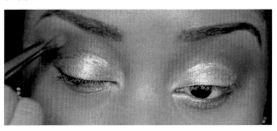

11. Apply eyeliner to top and bottom as well as mascara (or false lashes!)! I added a little glitter to my lid as well but you can leave out the glitter!

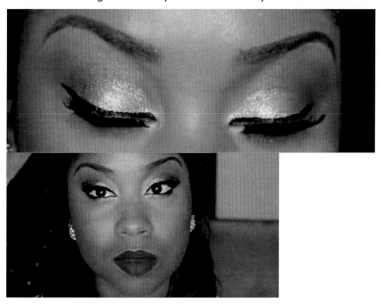

Awake eye shadow look

This is a great eye shadow look when you want to look awake. I highly recommend a smudge brush for this eye shadow look as the more blended, the better. You will need two eye shadow colors and an eyeliner pencil. I recommend the lighter shadow being pearl, satin or shimmer that is white, light pink or light beige.

1. Apply lightest eye shadow to your tear ducts and ½ of your waterline (inner)

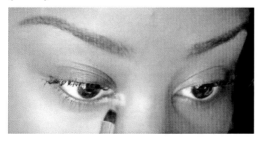

2. Take an eye pencil and line your waterline ½ of the way (outer)

33

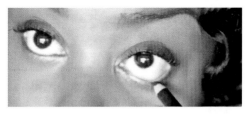

3. Take a dark eye shadow color and smudge out the eye pencil, making sure to not go over the light highlight eye shadow.

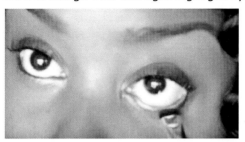

4. Apply mascara to the top and bottom lashes

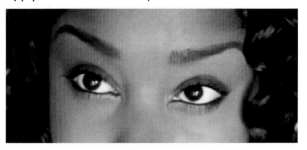

Eye shadow Brushes

You wouldn't paint a room in a house without the proper brushes, and nor do you want to apply your makeup without the proper tools! Makeup brushes can be overwhelming because this is so many brands and types on the market but as a beginner you only need a few until you are comfortable enough to explore more. Your makeup will drastically improve with the right brushes so I recommend playing around with brushes to get a good feel. The ones below are ones I really, really (no, really!) recommend for eye looks:

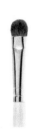

All-over Eye shadow Brush: Flat brush to apply eye shadow to lid and brow bone.
How to Use: Smooth eye shadow on your eyelid by packing it on.

Blending Brush: Used to blend out eye shadow for a soft blended look. Can also be used to apply color to your crease. How to Use: Hold the tip of the handle and swirl in a circular motions or windshield wiper motions.

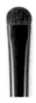

Smudge Brush: Line your waterline or lash line. Also great at smudging out pencil for a smoky look.
How to Use Sweep the brush side to side to create a smoky look.

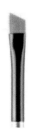

Angled Eyeliner Brush: Perfect for anything that needs a straight edge. Apply your eyebrow powder to brows, apply cream/gel liner to lash line and highlight tear duct.

How to use: hold the brush at an angle and allow bristles to brag from one side to the next.

Crease Brush: I especially recommend for those with deep set eyes or small eyes as it allows you to directly place eye shadow into your crease.

How to use: Dip in color and apply directly to crease. Wipe back and forth (windshield wiper motions)

Eyeliner

One of the most common questions I receive is how to apply eyeliner. With so many types (liquid, gel/crème, pencil, marker, and even eye shadow) I understand how a Girl (or boy!) can be overwhelmed! Before I start off this chapter, let me say that practice makes perfect! Seriously! It amazes me when people say they can't get the hang of liquid eyeliner and have literally applied it once. Pros were once amateurs so respect the process! I recommend taking a night (not the night of a big event!) but just taking a nice to play in makeup. I became good at makeup because I enjoyed playing and practicing in it. Instead of sitting on the couch watching TV, take that time and play in your makeup. Practice blending eye shadow, practice using eyeliner with an angled brush. Practice using tools, practice using methods. I cannot stress this enough. PRACTICE! *Whew* okay, now that I got off my chest, let's proceed!

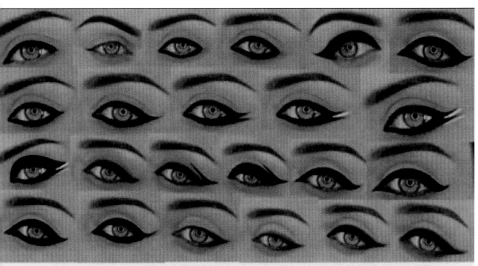

23 DIFFERENT EYELINER STYLES

Photo Credit: Maya Mia, https://www.youtube.com/user/007MayaMi

Different Types of Eyeliner

Liquid Eyeliner- liquid applied with a brush/application to create a sharp, precise line. Generally used to apply to upper lash line as it can be thick and heavy. Can be difficult for those with shaky hands.

How to Use:

1. Remove excess liquid by running the application on the edge of bottle
2. Starting from the center of your eye, draw short dashes to the outer corn of your eye.
3. Without adding more liquid to your brush, draw a short dash from your inner eye to the center of your eye
4. Connect your lid from the inner, center and outer

NOTE: If liquid is still too hard for you. I recommend applying small dots across your upper lash line. Then go in and connect those dots.

Pencil Eyeliner- Line your lids in pencil form. Generally easy to apply as it's just like writing with a pencil. However, is more likely to smudge. This can be a good thing if you want to smudge it out a smoky look.

How to Use:

1. Make sure your pencil is sharp (there are sharpeners made just for eye/lip pencils). Sharpening your pencil helps to remove any old bacteria from the pencil as well
2. Start from the inner corner of your eye and draw a dash ending at the center of your lid
3. From the center of your lid, draw a dash to the outer corner of your lid
4. Make sure the line is completely connected, smooth out line if needed.

Note: The difference between regular pencil liner and Kohl liner is that Kohl tends to glide on smoother (waxier). Great for those who want a smoother line or intense color.

Gel/Cream Eyeliner - eyeliner in a cream/gel form. Great for cat-eyes and intense color. Generally lost wearing and smudge-proof once dry. Can be difficult for those with shaky hands

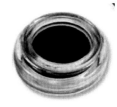

How to Use:

1. I recommend picking an eyeliner brush that works best for you. I personally prefer an angled brush or my personal favorite, the angled eyeliner brush. Make sure the brush is dense so you can draw a precise line. Before applying eyeliner, you want to make sure your brush is clean.
2. Dip brush lightly into gel/cream. Remember the great thing about gel liner is that it's buildable. You can always apply more!
3. Draw your tail at the outer edge of your eye
4. Now from the center of your eye, draw a line from the center of your lash line to the tail (should connect)
5. From your inner eye, draw a line to the center (should connect with the center liner)
6. Now smooth out line entirely

Recommended Brushes:

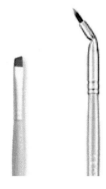

Pen: Liquid eyeliner in a pen. Great for those who want that liquid look but have not mastered it with the liquid

application. Takes a steady hand and pens tend to try out easily.

How to Use:

(See liquid eyeliner on how to use as the method is the same)

Shadow- Generally won't last as long as other eyeliner options. Does not work well on lower lash line but great for a subtle look.

How To Use:

(See gel eyeliner on how to use as the method is the same)

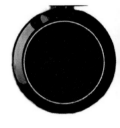

<u>Tips:</u>

- Apply eyeliner is small strokes. You can always make your line thicker but it's not nearly as easy to make it thinner

Mascara

Curling your Lashes:

Curling your lashes is a great way to help your eyelashes look fuller and longer. A good eyelash curler will lift your lashes, causing your eyes to appear more open.

Curly lashes (optional)

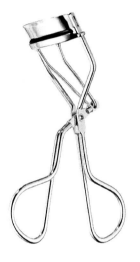

1. Hold the curler like you would normally hold a pair of scissors.
2. Open the curler completely and bring it to your upper lashes. You want to make sure to get the strip right up to the root of the eyelashes.
3. Ensure all of your lashes are inside the curler and no skin is inside your lashes.
4. Close the curler carefully on the lashes and squeeze lightly (should not hurt!), with a soft, pulsing grip.
5. Now turn the curler upwards to curl lashes
6. Now apply mascara!

Note:

You can heat your eyelash curler prior to curling lashes by applying heat to it for a few seconds with a hair dryer. Be sure the curler is not hot (should be warm) as this can burn lash hair or worst, your eye.

How to apply mascara

Tilt your head back so you the roots to your lashes are visible. Look straight forward. Take your mascara and apply from the root to the tip. I like to apply from the center first, then outer lashes and lastly my inner lashes. To elongate lashes, try rotating your mascara wand and sweeping upward through your lashes.

When applying mascara to your bottom lashes, tilt your head slightly forward so your roots on your bottom lashes are visible. Use side motions as you coat your bottom lashes with mascara to prevent getting mascara on your cheeks

Tips:

- Don't pump the want in and out. As this causes air to be pushed in the tube and dry out your mascara inside quicker
- Waterproof mascara is great for long wear as it has serious staying-power. It's a little harder to remove so I recommend dipping a q-tip in makeup remove and lightly gliding it on your bottom water line/lash line to remove water-proof mascara at night.
- Different Mascara wands do different things. Know that not all mascaras are made equally!

Makeup Steps

1. **Eyebrows**
   - Fill in eyebrows

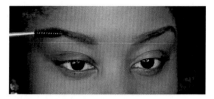

2. **Eye shadow Primer/Base**
   - Apply eye shadow primer and then eye shadow base (*note: some products combine both*)

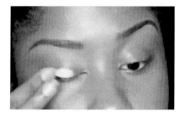

3. **Eye shadow**
   - Apply eye shadow

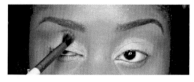

4. **Eyeliner**
   - Line eyes

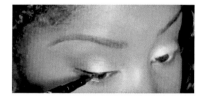

5. **Mascara (and/or Lashes)**
   a. Apply 2 coats of mascara to top and bottom lashes (optional: followed by fake lashes)

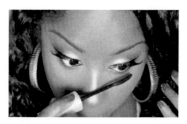

And there yam go! Be sure to check out the video tutorial for this look here: https://youtu.be/9l4ml-JDUgE

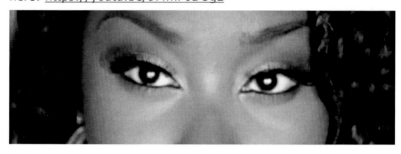